The Complete Guide to Air Fried Poultry Recipes

Time Saving and Effortless Recipes for Every Poultry Meal Lover

Tabitha Herring

contained within this document, including, but not limited to, — errors, omissions, or inaccuracies.

Table of contents

BBQ Chicken – Gluten-Free

Serves:4

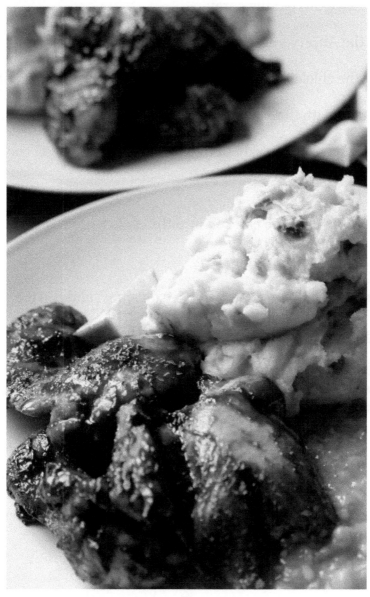

- Boneless – skinless chicken breast (2 large)
- Seasoned flour/Gluten-free seasoned flour (.5 cup)

  Barbecue sauce (1 cup)
- Olive oil cooking spray

1. Heat the Air Fryer to 390° Fahrenheit.

2. Chop the chicken into bite-size chunks and place in a mixing bowl. Coat with the seasoned flour.

3. Lightly spritz the basket of the Air Fryer with olive oil cooking spray

4. and evenly pour the chicken into the cooker.

5. Set the timer for 8 minutes.

6. Open the Air Fryer, coat with olive oil spray, and flip the chicken as needed.

7. Air-fry the chicken for eight more minutes.

8. Be sure its internal reading is at least 165° Fahrenheit.

9. Place the chicken into a dish and add the sauce to cover. Line the Air Fryer with a sheet of foil or add the chicken back to the fryer and cook for another 3 minutes until the sauce is warmed

and the chicken is a bit more crispy and coated. Serve.

Buffalo Chicken Wings

Serves:2-3

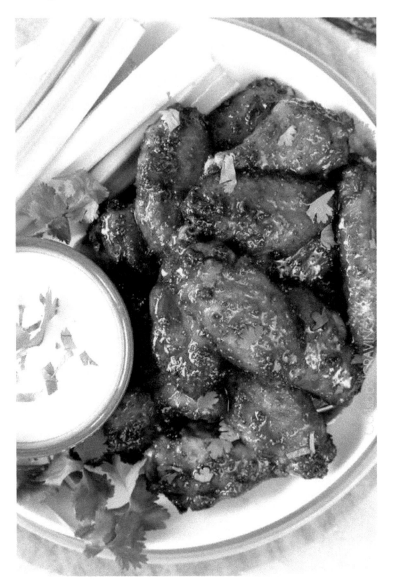

- Chicken wings (5 – trombo. 14 oz.)

- Salt & black pepper (as desired)

- Cayenne pepper (2 tsp. or to taste)

- Red hot sauce (2 tbsp.)

- Melted butter (1 tbsp.)

- Optional: Garlic powder (.5 tsp.)

- Heat the Air Fryer temperature to reach 356° Fahrenheit.

- Slice the wings into three sections (end tip, middle joint, and drumstick). Pat each one thoroughly dry using a paper towel.

- Combine the pepper, salt, garlic powder, and cayenne pepper on a platter. Lightly cover the wings with the powder.

- Arrange the chicken onto the wire rack and bake for 15 minutes, turning once at 7 minutes.

- Combine the hot sauce with the melted butter in a dish to garnish the baked chicken when it is time to be served.

Chicken Breast Tenderloins

Serves: 4

- Butter/vegetable oil (2 tbsp.)

- Breadcrumbs (3.33 tbsp.)

- Egg (1)

- Chicken tenderloins (8)

1. Heat the Air Fryer temperature to 356° Fahrenheit.

2. Combine the breadcrumbs and oil – stirring until the mixture crumbles.

3. Whisk the egg and dredge the chicken through the egg, shaking off the excess.

4. Dip each piece of chicken into the crumbs and evenly coat.

5. Set the timer for 12 minutes.

Chicken Curry

Serves:4

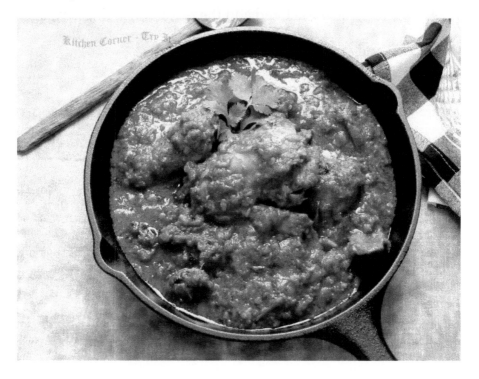

- Chicken breast (1 lb.) Olive oil (1 tsp.) Onion (1)

- Garlic (2 tsp.)

- Lemongrass (1 tbsp.) Chicken stock (.5 cup)

- Apple cider vinegar (1 tbsp.) Coconut milk (.5 cup)

- Curry paste (2 tbsp.)

- Warm the fryer to reach 365° Fahrenheit.

- Dice the chicken into cubes. Peel and dice the onion and combine in the Air Fryer basket. Cook for five minutes.
- Remove the basket and add the rest of the fixings. Mix well and air- fry for ten more minutes.
- Serve for a quick and easy meal.

Chicken Fillet Strips

Serves:4

- Chicken fillets (1 lb.)

- Paprika (1 tsp.)

- Heavy cream (1 tbsp.)

- Salt & pepper (.5 tsp.) Butter (as needed)

- Heat the Air Fryer at 365° Fahrenheit.

- Slice the fillets into strips and dust with salt and pepper.

- Add a light coating of butter to the basket.

- Arrange the strips in the basket and air-fry for six minutes.

- Flip the strips and continue frying for another five minutes.

- When done, garnish with the cream and paprika. Serve warm.

Chicken Kabobs

Serves: 2

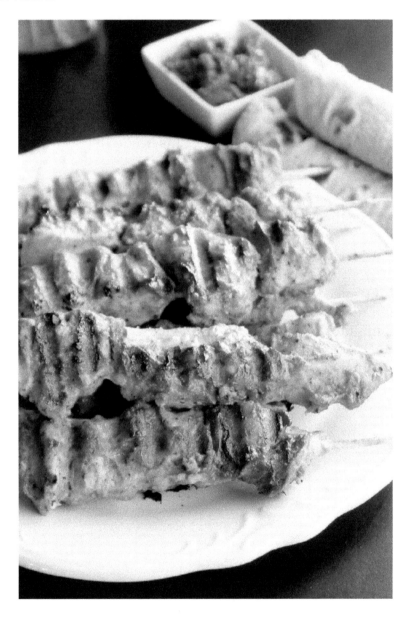

- Chicken breasts (2) Mushrooms (6)

- Bell peppers (3 various colors)

- Honey (.33 cup) Soy sauce (.33 cup)

- Salt and pepper (to your liking) Sesame seeds

- Set the temperature of the fryer to 338° Fahrenheit.

- Slice the mushrooms in half. Dice the peppers and chicken.

- Coat the chicken with a couple of squirts of oil and a pinch of pepper and salt.

- Mix the soy and honey. Toss in a few sesame seeds and stir.

- Arrange the peppers, chicken, and mushroom bits onto a skewer.

- Cover the kabobs with the sauce and arrange them in the basket of the Air Fryer.

- Air-fry for 15-20 minutes and serve.

Chicken Pot Pie

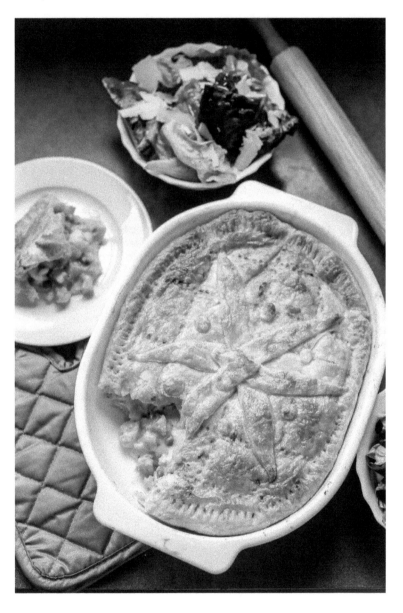

- Chicken tenders (6)

- Potatoes (2)
- Condensed cream of celery soup (1.5 cups) Heavy cream (.75 cup)
- Thyme (1 sprig)
- Dried bay leaf (1 whole) Refrigerated buttermilk biscuits (5) Milk (1 tbsp.)
- Egg yolk (1)

1.Set the Air Fryer at 320° Fahrenheit.

2.Peel and dice the potatoes. Combine all of the fixings in a skillet except for the milk, egg yolk, and biscuits. Bring it to a boil using the medium-heat temperature setting.

3.Empty the mixture into the baking tin. Cover with a sheet of aluminum foil. Prepare a sling using a length of foil to make a handle. Place the pan into the fry basket using the sling and cook for 15 minutes.

4.After the pie completes the cycle, prepare an egg wash using the milk and egg yolk.

5.Arrange the biscuits onto the baking pan and brush using the egg wash mixture. Set the timer for an additional ten minutes (300° Fahrenheit).

6.Serve when the biscuits are golden brown.

Crispy Chicken Sliders

Serves: 6

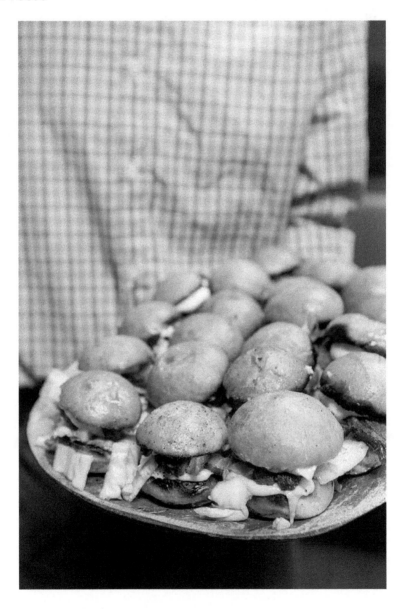

- Tyson Crispy Chicken Strips (1 pkg.)

- Sweet Hawaiian Rolls (1 pkg.)

- Optional: Spinach leaves Tomatoes Honey mustard

- Place the six chicken strips in the Air Fryer basket with a coating of olive oil spray. Cook at 390° Fahrenheit for 8 minutes.

- Slice the rolls in half and top them with honey mustard, spinach, and tomatoes or other toppings of your choice.

- Slice the chicken strips into chunks and place them on the rolls.

Fried Chicken Thighs

Serves: 2

- Chicken thighs – no skin (2)

- Fresh parsley (3 sprigs) Garlic powder – for dusting
  Lemon (half if 1)

- Fresh rosemary (1-2 sprigs)

- Chili flakes – salt & black pepper (as desired)

1.Rinse the thighs and drain between a few paper towels.

2.Clean the rosemary sprigs and remove the stems. Mince the

parsley.

3.Combine the parsley, chili flakes, salt, pepper, garlic

powder, rosemary leaves, and lemon juice. Add the thighs and

marinate overnight in the fridge.

4.Warm the Air Fryer at 356⁰ Fahrenheit. Air-fry for 12 minutes.

Garlic Herb Turkey Breast

Serves: 6

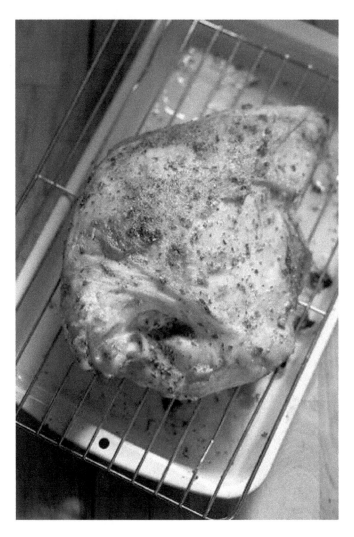

- Turkey breast (2 lb.)

- Freshly ground black pepper & Kosher salt Melted butter
  (4 tbsp.)

- Garlic (3 cloves)

- Thyme (1 tsp.)

- Rosemary (1 tsp.)

- Warm the Air Fryer to reach 375° Fahrenheit.

- Pat the turkey breast dry and season both sides with salt and pepper.

- Mince the garlic and chop the rosemary and thyme.

- In a small bowl, combine the melted butter, garlic, thyme, and rosemary. Brush using butter all over turkey breast.

- Place in the Air Fryer basket, skin side up, and cook for 40 minutes

- or until internal temperature reaches 160° Fahrenheit, flipping halfway through.

- Wait for five minutes before slicing.

Mustard-Glazed Turkey Breast

Serves: 6

- Olive oil (2 tsp.)

- Whole turkey breast (5 lb.) Salt (1 tsp.)

- Dried thyme (1 tsp.) Butter (1 tsp.)

- Freshly cracked black pepper (.5 tsp.) Smoked paprika (.5 tsp.)

- Dried sage (.5 tsp.) Maple syrup (.25 tsp.) Dijon mustard (2 tbsp.)

- Warm the fryer to 350° Fahrenheit.

- Prepare the turkey with a spritz of olive oil.

- Mix the sage, salt, thyme, pepper, and paprika as a rub. Use it as a coating for the turkey.

- Arrange the breast in the fryer basket and set the timer for 25 minutes. Rotate it on its side and fry another 12 minutes. It's done when it reaches 165° Fahrenheit – internal temperature.

- In the meantime, whisk the butter, syrup, and mustard in a saucepan. Turn the breast again and brush using the glaze. Give it a final five minutes until crispy.
- Cover using a foil tent for five minutes, slice, and serve.

Parmesan Chicken

Serves:4

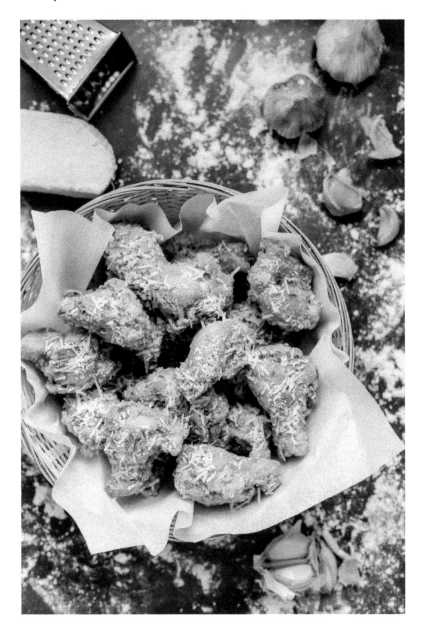

- Chicken breast (2 – about 8 oz. each)

- Seasoned breadcrumbs (6 tbsp.)

- Grated parmesan cheese (2 tbsp.)

- Olive oil/melted butter (1 tbsp.)

- Reduced-fat mozzarella cheese (6 tbsp.)

- Marinara sauce (.5 cup)

1.Set the Air Fryer at 360° Fahrenheit for 3 minutes.

2.Slice the chicken breasts into halves, then into four thin cutlets.

3.Combine the parmesan cheese and breadcrumbs in a bowl.

4.Melt the butter in another dish.

5.Lightly brush the butter onto the chicken, then dip into the breadcrumb mixture.

6.When the Air Fryer is ready, arrange two pieces in the basket and spray the top with a bit of cooking oil.

7. Fry for 6 minutes; turn and top each with one tablespoon of the sauce, and 1.5 tablespoons of shredded mozzarella cheese.

8.Cook until the cheese is melted (3 min.).

9.Set aside and keep warm, repeat with the remaining two
pieces.

Philly Chicken Cheese Steak Stromboli

Serves: 2-4

- Vegetable oil (1 tsp.) Onion (half of 1)

- Chicken breasts (2/total of 1 lb.) Worcestershire sauce (1 tbsp.)

- Pizza dough (14 oz. pkg. – homemade or store-bought) Freshly cracked black pepper & salt

- Cheese Whiz or your favorite cheese sauce (.5 cup) Grated Cheddar cheese (1.5 cups)

- Warm the Cheese Whiz in the microwave.

- Set the temperature to 400° Fahrenheit in the Air Fryer.

- Place the onion in the fryer for eight minutes – shaking gently halfway through the cycle. Thinly slice and add the chicken and Worcestershire sauce, salt, and pepper – tossing evenly. Air fry for another eight minutes – stirring several times. Remove and let the mixture cool.

- Lightly flour a flat surface and press out the dough into a rectangle of 11x13 (the long side facing you). Sprinkle half

of the cheddar over the dough. Leave a one-inch border –
topping it off with the onion/chicken mixture.

- Drizzle the warmed cheese sauce over the top, finishing
  with the rest of the cheddar cheese.

- Roll the tromboli toward the empty corner (away from
  you). Keep the filling tight and tuck in the ends. Arrange
  it seam side down and shape in a "U" to fit into the
  basket. Slice four slits in the top with the tip of a knife.

- Lightly brush the top with a little oil. Set the temperature
  to 370° Fahrenheit.

- Spray the basket and add the stromboli. Fry for 12
  minutes – turning about halfway through the cooking
  process.

- Use a serving platter and invert the tasty treat from the
  basket. Arrange it on a cutting board and cut into three-
  inch segments. Serve with ketchup for dipping.

Chicken Tenders

Serves: 4

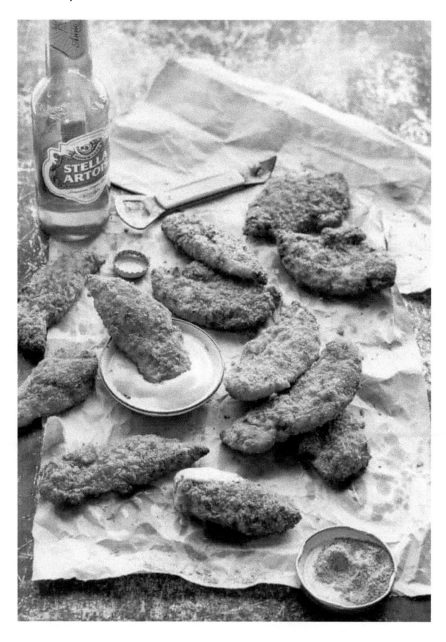

- 1lb. Chicken tenders 1 egg, lightly beaten

- 3/4 cup pecans, crushed

- ¼ cup ground mustard

- ½ tsp paprika

- tsp garlic powder

- ¼ tsp onion powder 1/4 tsp pepper

- 1 tsp salt

1.Spray air fryer basket with cooking spray.

2.Add chicken into the large bowl. Season with paprika, pepper, garlic powder, onion powder, and salt. Add mustard mix well.

3.In a separate bowl, add egg and whisk well.

4.In a shallow bowl, add crushed pecans.

5.Dip chicken into the egg then coats with pecans and place into the air fryer basket.

6.Cook at 350 f for 12 minutes.

7.Serve and enjoy.

CHICKEN COCONUT MEATBALLS

Servings: 4

- 1lb. Ground chicken 1 ½ tsp sriracha

- 1/2 tbsp soy sauce 1/2 tbsp hoisin sauce

- ¼ cup shredded coconut 1 tsp sesame oil

- ½ cup fresh cilantro, chopped

- 1 green onions, 1 chopped Pepper

- Salt

1.Spray air fryer basket with cooking spray.

2.Add all into the large bowl and mix until well combined.

3.Make small balls from meat mixture and place into the air fryer basket.

4.Cook at 350 f for 10 minutes. Turn halfway through.

5.Serve and enjoy.

Cheese Herb Chicken Wings

Servings: 4

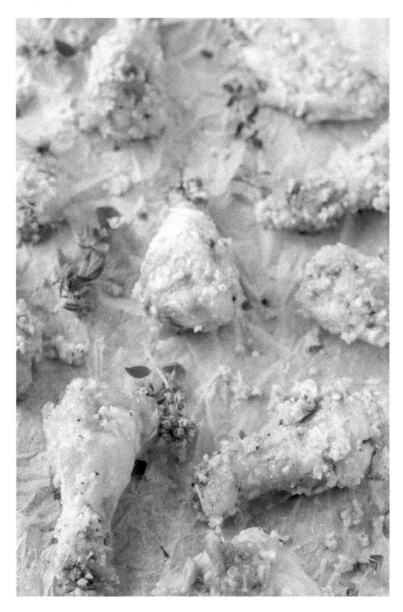

- 2lbs. Chicken wings

- 1 tsp herb de provence

- ½ cup parmesan cheese, grated 1 tsp paprika

- Salt

1.Preheat the air fryer to 350 f.

2. In a small bowl, mix cheese, herb de provence, paprika, and salt.

3.Spray air fryer basket with cooking spray.

4.Toss chicken wings with cheese mixture and place into the air fryer basket and cook for 15 minutes. Turn halfway through.

5.Serve and enjoy.

Delicious Chicken Tenderloins

Serves: 6

- egg, lightly beaten
- ¼ cup heavy whipping cream 8 oz chicken breast tenderloins 1 cup almond flour
- ¼ tsp garlic powder
- ¼ tsp onion powder 1 tsp pepper
- tsp salt
- Whisk egg, with garlic powder, onion powder, cream, pepper, and salt in a bowl.
- In a shallow dish, add the almond flour.
- Dip chicken in egg mixture then coats with almond flour mixture.
- Spray air fryer basket with cooking spray.
- Place chicken into the air fryer basket and cook at 450 f for 15 minutes.
- Serve and enjoy.

GARLIC HERB CHICKEN BREASTS

Serves: 5

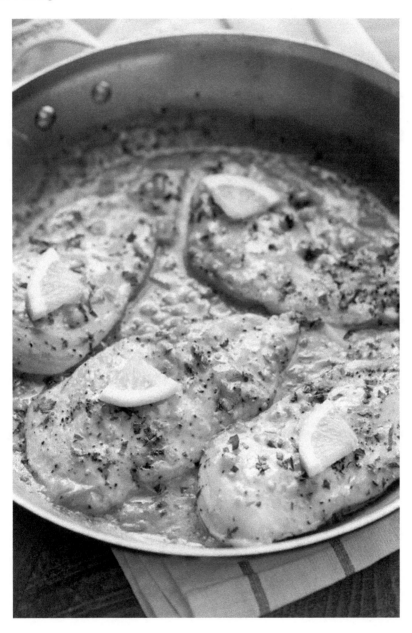

- 2lbs. Chicken breasts, skinless and boneless
- 2garlic cloves, minced
- ¼ cup yogurt
- ¼ cup mayonnaise
- 2 tsp garlic herb seasoning 1/2 tsp onion powder
- ¼ tsp salt
- Preheat the air fryer to 380 f.
- In a small bowl, mix mayonnaise, seasoning, onion powder, garlic, and yogurt.
- Brush chicken with mayo mixture and season with salt.
- Spray air fryer basket with cooking spray.
- Place chicken into the air fryer basket and cook for 15 minutes.
- Serve and enjoy.

Tasty Caribbean Chicken

Serves: 8

- 3lbs. Chicken thigh, skinless and boneless 1 tbsp coriander powder
- 3 tbsp coconut oil, melted
- ½ tsp ground nutmeg
- ½ tsp ground ginger 1 tbsp cayenne
- 1 tbsp cinnamon
- Pepper and salt
- In a small bowl, mix all spices and rub all over the chicken.
- Spray air fryer basket with cooking spray.
- Place chicken into the air fryer basket and cook at 390 f for 10 minutes.
- Serve and enjoy.

CHICKEN KABAB

Servings: 3

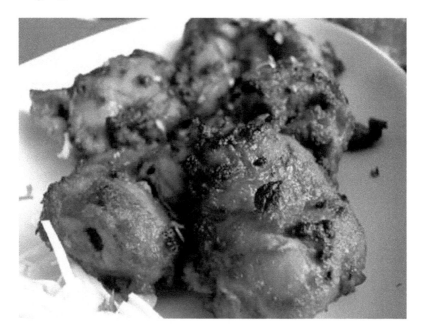

- lb. Ground chicken

- tbsp fresh lemon juice

- ¼ cup almond flour

- green onion, chopped 1 egg, lightly beaten

- 1/3 cup fresh parsley, chopped 3 garlic cloves

- oz onion, chopped

- ¼ tsp turmeric powder

- ½ tsp pepper

1.Add all into the food processor and process until well combined.

2.Transfer chicken mixture to the bowl and place in the refrigerator for 1 hour.

3.Divide mixture into the 6 equal portions and roll around the soaked wooden skewers.

4. Spray air fryer basket with cooking spray.

5.Place skewers into the air fryer basket and cooks at 400 f for 6 minutes.

6.Serve and enjoy.

Mediterranean Chicken

Servings: 6

- lbs. Whole chicken, cut into pieces 2 tsp ground sumac

- 2 garlic cloves, minced 2 lemons, sliced

- 2 tbsp olive oil 1 tsp lemon zest 2 tsp kosher salt

1.Rub chicken with oil, sumac, lemon zest, and salt. Place in the refrigerator for 2-3 hours.

2.Add lemon sliced into the air fryer basket top with marinated chicken.

3.Cook at 350 for 35 minutes.

4.Serve and enjoy.

Asian Chicken Wings

Servings: 2

- chicken wings
- 3/4 tbsp chinese spice 1 tbsp soy sauce
- tsp mixed spice Pepper
- Salt

1.Add chicken wings into the bowl. Add remaining and toss to coat.

2.Transfer chicken wings into the air fryer basket.

3.Cook at 350 f for 15 minutes.

4.Turn chicken to another side and cook for 15 minutes more.

5.Serve and enjoy.

Delicious Chicken Fajitas

Servings: 4

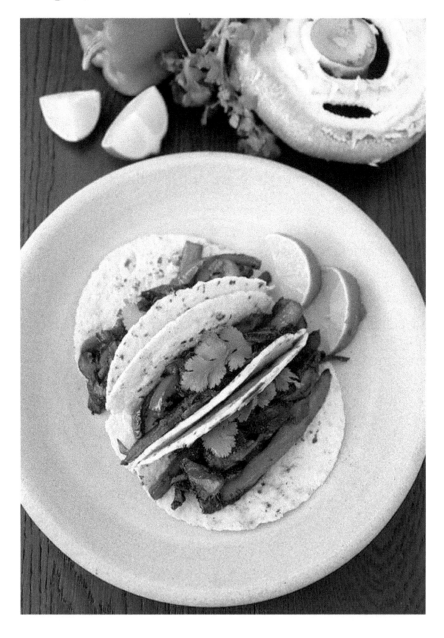

- chicken breasts

- onion, sliced

- bell pepper, sliced

- 1 1/2 tbsp fajita seasoning 2 tbsp olive oil

- 3/4 cup cheddar cheese, shredded

- Preheat the air fryer at 380 f.

- Coat chicken with oil and rub with seasoning.

- Place chicken into the air fryer baking dish and top with bell peppers and onion.

- Cook for 15 minutes.

- Top with shredded cheese and cook for 1-2 minutes until cheese is melted.

- Serve and enjoy.

Juicy & Spicy Chicken Wings

Servings: 4

- lbs. Chicken wings 12 oz hot sauce

- tsp worcestershire sauce

- tsp tabasco

- tbsp butter, melted

- Spray air fryer basket with Cooking spray.

- Add chicken wings into the air fryer basket and cook at 380 f for 25 minutes. Shake basket after every 5 minutes.

- Meanwhile, in a bowl, mix hot sauce, worcestershire sauce, and butter. Set aside.

- Add chicken wings into the sauce and toss well.

- Serve and enjoy.

Indian Chicken Tenders

Servings: 4

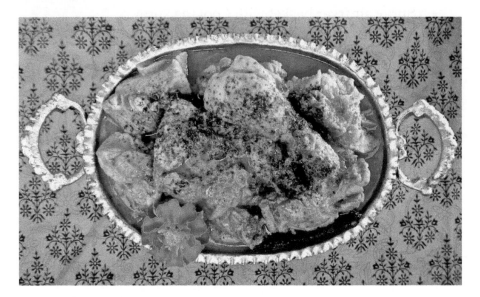

1. 1lb. Chicken tenders, cut in half

2. ¼ cup parsley, chopped

3. 1/2 tbsp garlic, minced

4. 1/2 tbsp ginger, minced

5. ¼ cup yogurt 3/4 tsp paprika

6. 1 tsp garam masala 1 tsp turmeric

7. 1/2 tsp cayenne pepper 1 tsp salt

- Preheat the air fryer to 350 f.

- Add all into the large bowl and mix well. Place in refrigerator for 30 minutes.
- Spray air fryer basket with Cooking spray.
- Add marinated chicken into the air fryer basket and cook for 10 minutes.
- Turn chicken to another side and cook for 5 minutes more.
- Serve and enjoy.

Dijon Turkey Drumstick

Servings: 2

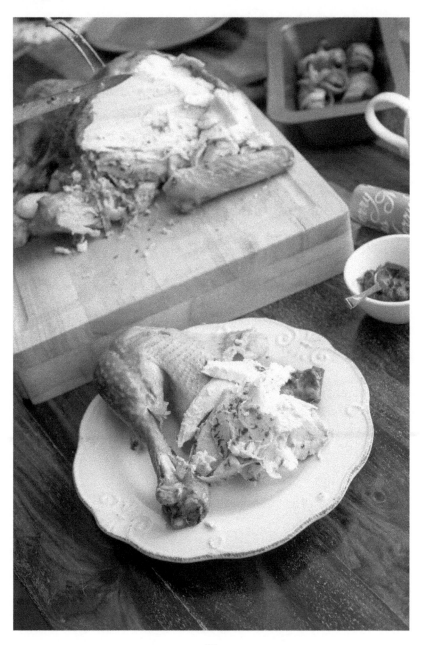

- 4 turkey drumsticks
- 1/3 tsp paprika
- 1/3 cup sherry wine
- 1/3 cup coconut milk
- 1/2 tbsp ginger, minced
- 2 tbsp dijon mustard Pepper
- Salt

- Add all Ingredients into the large bowl and stir to coat. Place in refrigerator for 2 hours.
- Spray air fryer basket with cooking spray.
- Place marinated turkey drumsticks into the air fryer basket and cook at 380 f for 28 minutes. Turn halfway through.
- Serve and enjoy.

Curried Drumsticks

Servings: 2

- 2 turkey drumsticks
- 1/3 cup coconut milk
- 1/2 tbsp ginger, minced
- 1/4 tsp cayenne pepper
- 1/4 tbsp red curry paste
- 1/4 tsp pepper
- 1/4 tsp kosher salt
- Add all into the bowl and stir to coat. Place in refrigerator for overnight.
- Spray air fryer basket with cooking spray.
- Place marinated drumsticks into the air fryer basket and cook at 390 f for 22 minutes.
- Serve and enjoy.

Korean Chicken Tenders

Servings: 3

- 12 oz chicken tenders, skinless and boneless
- 2 tbsp green onion, chopped 3 garlic cloves, chopped
- 2 tsp sesame seeds, toasted
- 1 tbsp ginger, grated
- 1/4 cup sesame oil
- 1/2 cup soy sauce
- 1/4 tsp pepper
- Slide chicken tenders onto the skewers.
- In a large bowl, mix green onion, garlic, sesame seeds, ginger, sesame oil, soy sauce, and pepper.
- Add chicken skewers into the bowl and coat well with marinade.
- Place in refrigerator for overnight.
- Preheat the air fryer to 390 f.
- Place marinated chicken skewers into the air fryer basket and cook for 10 minutes.

Air Fried Chicken With Coconut & Turmeric

Servings: 3

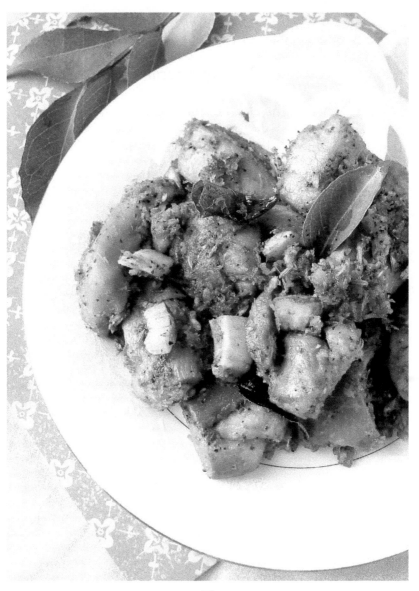

- 1½ oz. Coconut milk

- 3 tsp. Ginger, grated

- 4 tsp. Ground turmeric

- ½ tsp. Sea salt

- 3 chicken legs (skin removed)

1.Combine the coconut milk, ginger, turmeric and salt.

2.Make a few slits on the chicken meat.

3.Marinate the chicken in the mixture for 4 hours.

4.Keep inside the refrigerator.

5.Preheat air fryer at 375 degrees f.

6.Cook for 10 minutes.

7.Flip and cook for another 10 to 12 minutes.

Chicken Parmesan

Servings: 4

- 1 egg

- 1 tsp. Garlic powder 1 tsp. Italian herbs

- 8 breast-meat chicken tenders

- ½ cup parmesan cheese

- 1 cup panko breadcrumbs

1.Beat the egg in a bowl.

2.Add the garlic powder and italian herbs.

3.Soak the chicken strips in this mixture.

4.In a different bowl, mix the parmesan and breadcrumbs.

5.Coat the chicken tenders with the parmesan mixture.

6.Cover the air fryer base with foil.

7.Preheat at 400 degrees f for 3 minutes.

8. Put the chicken tenders inside the basket.

9.Cook for 6 minutes.

10.Serve while warm.

Crunchy Curry Chicken Strips

Servings: 4

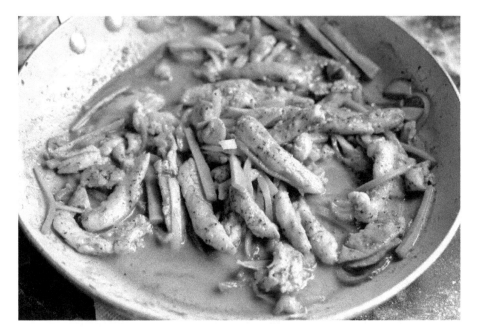

- 12 oz. Chicken breast, cut into strips

- Salt and pepper to taste

- 1 egg, beaten

- ¼ cup whole wheat flour

- ½ cup panko breadcrumbs

- ¼ cup curry powder

- Season the chicken strips with the salt and pepper.

- Dip each of the chicken strips into the flour, then into the egg.

- In a bowl, mix the curry powder and breadcrumbs.

- Coat each of the chicken strips with the curry powder mixture.

- Cook in the air fryer at 350 degrees f for 10 minutes.

- Flip and cook for another 5 minutes.

Chicken Pie

Servings: 8 to 10

- 2 chicken thighs (boneless, sliced into cubes)

- 1 tsp. Reduced Sodium soy sauce

- 1 onion, diced

- 1 carrot, diced

- 2 potatoes, diced

- 1 cup mushrooms

- 1 tsp. Garlic powder 1 tsp. Flour½ cup milk

- **2** hard-boiled eggs, sliced in half 2 sheets puff pastry

1.Season the chicken cubes with the low Sodium soy sauce.

2.In a pan over low heat, sauté the onions, carrots and potatoes.

3.Add the chicken cubes and mushrooms.

4.Season with the garlic powder.

5.Add the flour and milk.

6.Mix well.

7.Lay the pastry sheet on the tray of the air fryer.

8.Poke it with holes using a fork.

9.Arrange the eggs on top of the pastry sheet.

10.Pour in the chicken mixture on top of the eggs.

11.Top with the second pastry sheet.

12.Press a little.

13.Air fry at 360 degrees f for 6 minutes.

14.Slice into several portions and serve.

Buttermilk Chicken

Servings: 6 to 8

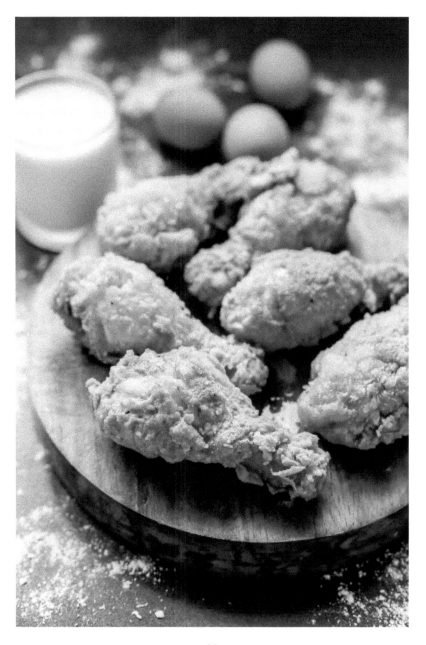

- 30 oz. Chicken thighs (skinless)
- 1 ½ tsp. salt
- 2 tsp. Black pepper
- 1 ½ tbsp. Garlic powder
- 2 cups buttermilk
- 2 cups all-purpose flour
- 1 tsp. Paprika powder
- 1 tbsp. Baking powder

1. Season the chicken with the salt, pepper and garlic powder.

2. Coat the chicken with the buttermilk.

3. Marinate in the refrigerator covered for 6 hours.

4. Preheat the air fryer at 360 degrees f.

5. In another bowl, mix the all-purpose flour, paprika powder and baking powder.

6. Dredge the chicken in this mixture.

7. Cook in the air fryer for 8 minutes.

8. Flip the chicken and cook for another 10 minutes.

9. Drain in paper towels before serving.

Lemon Chili Chicken Wings

Servings: 4

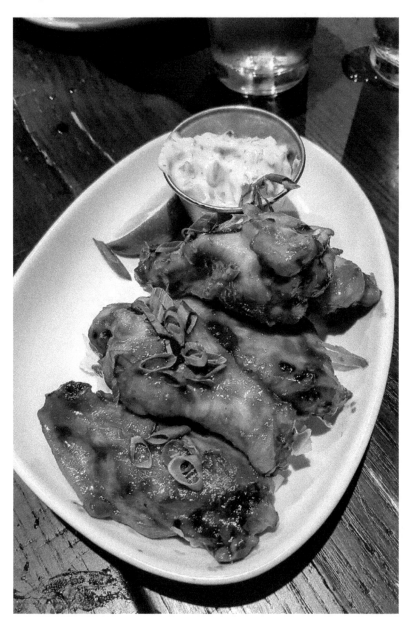

- 8 chicken wings

- Sea salt and pepper to taste 1 tbsp. Lemon juice

- 1 tbsp. Chili paste

- 2 tbsp. Cornstarch

- ½ tsp. Baking powder

- Rub the chicken wings with a little salt and pepper.

- Combine the lemon juice and chili paste.

- Soak the chicken wings in the chili mixture.

- Cover with foil and refrigerate for 4 hours.

- Preheat your air fryer to 360 degrees f.

- Coat the chicken wings with a mix of the cornstarch and baking powder.

- Air fry for 12 minutes.

- Flip and cook for another 6 minutes.

Lemon Garlic Rosemary Chicken

Servings: 2

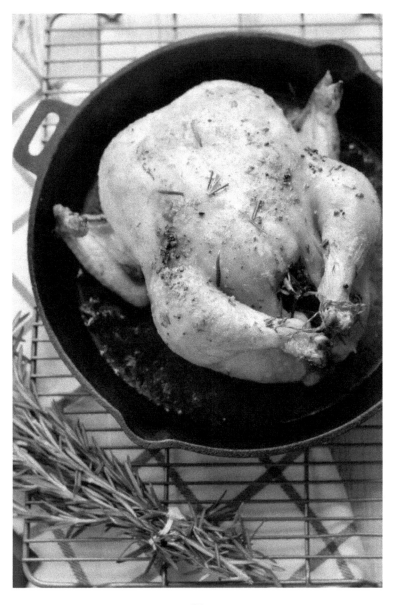

1.4 chicken thighs (skin removed)

2.Sea salt and pepper to taste

3.1 tbsp. Lemon juice

4.3 tsp. Dried rosemary

5.3 cloves garlic, crushed and minced

6.1 tsp. Olive oil

1.Season the chicken thighs with the sea salt, pepper, lemon juice, and dried rosemary.

2.Marinate for 1 hour.

3.Meanwhile, sauté the crushed garlic in the olive oil.

4.Cook the chicken thighs in the air fryer at 400 degrees for 6 minutes.

5.Flip the chicken and cook for another 6 minutes.

6.Pour the garlic oil on top of the chicken before serving.

Fried Whole Chicken

Servings: 4

- 1 whole chicken

- 2 tbsp or spray of oil of choice

- 1 tsp garlic powder

- 1 tsp onion powder

- 1 tsp paprika

- 1 tsp italian seasoning

- 2 tbsp montreal steak seasoning (or salt and pepper to taste)

- 1.4 cup chicken broth

- Truss and wash the chicken.

- Mix the seasoning and rub a little amount on the chicken.

- Pour the broth inside the instant pot duo crisp air fryer.

- Place the chicken in the air fryer basket.

- Select the option air fry and close the air fryer lid and cook for 25 minutes.

- Spray or rub the top of the chicken with oil and rub it with half of the seasoning.

- Close the air fryer lid and air fry again at 400°f for 10 minutes.

- Flip the chicken, spray it with oil, and rub with the remaining seasoning.

- Again, air fry it for another ten minutes.

- Allow the chicken to rest for 10 minutes.

Barbecue Air Fried Chicken

Servings: 10

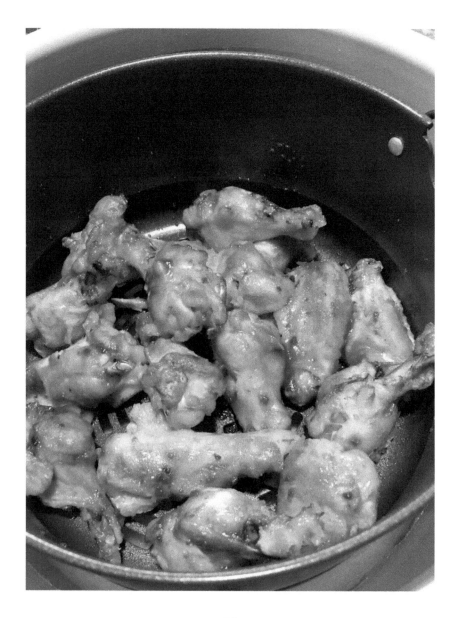

- 1 teaspoon liquid smoke

- 2 cloves fresh garlic smashed

- 1/2 cup apple cider vinegar

- 3 pounds chuck roast well-marbled with intramuscular Fat

- 1 tablespoon kosher salt

- 1 tablespoon freshly ground black pepper

- 2 teaspoons garlic powder

- 1.5 cups barbecue sauce

- 1/4 cup light brown Sugar + more for sprinkling

- tablespoons honey optional and in place of 2 tbl Sugar

- Add meat to the instant pot duo crisp air fryer basket, spreading out the meat.

- Select the option air fry.

- Close the air fryer lid and cook at 300 degrees f for 8 minutes. Pause the air fryer and flip meat over after 4 minutes.

- Remove the lid and baste with more barbecue sauce and sprinkle with a little brown Sugar.

- Again, close the air fryer lid and set the temperature at 400°f for 9 minutes. Watch meat though the lid and flip it over after 5 minutes.

Boneless Air Fryer Turkey Breasts

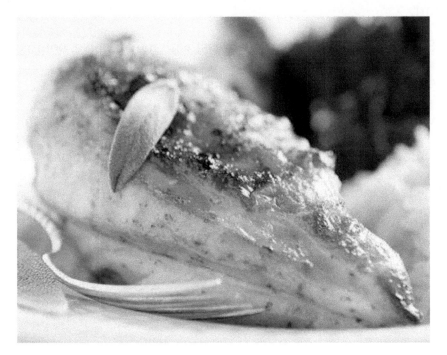

- 3 lb. Boneless breast

- ¼ cup mayonnaise

- 2 tsp poultry seasoning

- 1 tsp salt

- ½ tsp garlic powder

- ¼ tsp black pepper

1.Choose the air fry option on the instant pot duo crisp air fryer. Set the temperature to 360°f and push start. The preheating will start.

2.Season your boneless turkey breast with mayonnaise, poultry

3.seasoning, salt, garlic powder, and black pepper.

4.Once preheated, air fry the turkey breasts on 360°f for 1 hour, turning every 15 minutes or until internal temperature has reached a temperature of 165°f.

Bbq Chicken Breasts

Servings: 4

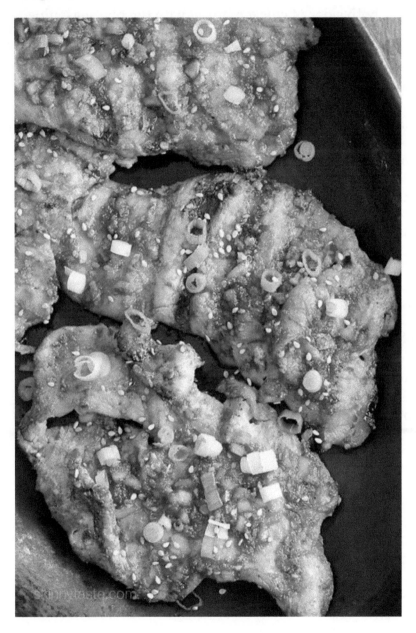

1.4 boneless skinless chicken breasts about 6 oz each

2.1-2 tbsp bbq seasoning

1.Cover both sides of chicken breast with the bbq seasoning. Cover and marinate the in the refrigerator for 45 minutes.

2.Choose the air fry option and set the temperature to 400°f. Push

3.start and let it preheat for 5 minutes.

4.Upon preheating, place the chicken breast in the instant pot duo crisp air fryer basket, making sure they do not overlap. Spray with oil.

5.Cook for 13-14 minutes, flipping halfway.

6.Remove chicken when the chicken reaches an internal temperature of 160°f. Place on a plate and allow to rest for 5 minutes before slicing.

Juicy Turkey Burgers

Servings: 8

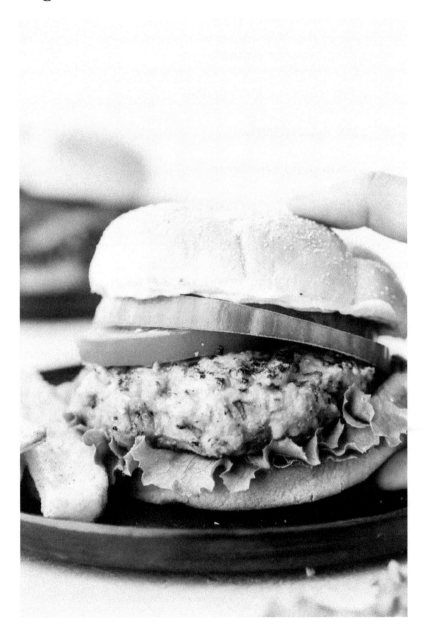

- 1 lb. Ground turkey 85% lean / 15% Fat

- ¼ cup unsweetened apple sauce

- ½ onion grated

- 1 tbsp ranch seasoning

- 2 tsp worcestershire sauce

- 1 tsp minced garlic

- ¼ cup plain breadcrumbs

- Salt and pepper to taste

- Combine the onion, ground turkey, unsweetened apple sauce, minced garlic, breadcrumbs, ranch seasoning, worchester sauce, and salt and pepper. Mix them with your hands until well combined. Form 4 equally sized hamburger patties with them.

- Place these burgers in the refrigerator for about 30 minutes to have them firm up a bit.

- While preparing for Cooking, select the air fry option. Set the temperature of 360°f and the cook time as required. Press start to

- begin preheating.

- Once the preheating temperature is reached, place the burgers on the tray in the air fryer basket, making sure they don't overlap or touch. Cook on for 15 minutes, flipping halfway through.

Turkey Legs

Servings: 2

- 2 large turkey legs

- 1 1/2 tsp smoked paprika

- 1 tsp brown Sugar

- 1 tsp season salt

- ½ tsp garlic powder

- Oil for spraying avocado, canola, etc.

1.Mix the smoked paprika, brown Sugar, seasoned salt, garlic powder thoroughly.

2.Wash and pat dry the turkey legs.

3.Rub the made seasoning mixture all over the turkey legs making sure to get under the skin also.

4.While preparing for Cooking, select the air fry option. Press start to begin preheating.

5.Once the preheating temperature is reached, place the turkey legs on the tray in the instant pot duo crisp air fryer basket. Lightly spray them with oil.

6.Air fry the turkey legs on 400°f for 20 minutes. Then, open the air fryer lid and flip the turkey legs and lightly spray with oil. Close

7.the instant pot duo crisp air fryer lid and cook for 20 more minutes.

8.Remove and enjoy.

Zingy & Nutty Chicken Wings

Servings: 4

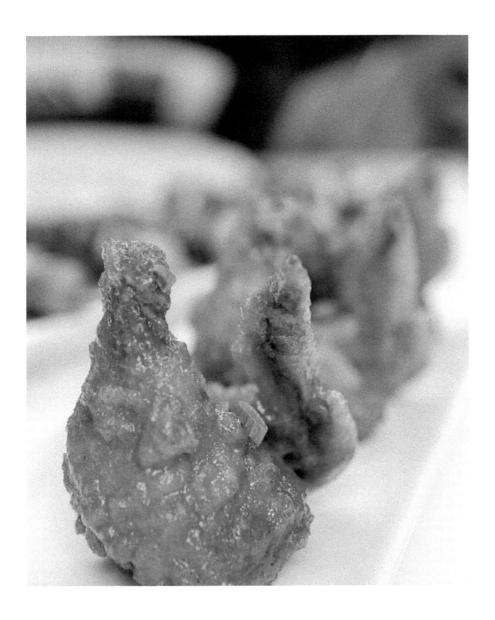

- 1 tablespoon fish sauce

- 1 tablespoon fresh lemon juice

- 1 teaspoon Sugar

- 12 chicken middle wings, cut into half

- 2 fresh lemongrass stalks, chopped finely

- ¼ cup unsalted cashews, crushed

1.In a bowl, mix fish sauce, lime juice and Sugar.

2.Add wings ad coat with mixture generously. Refrigerate to marinate for about 1-2 hours.

3.Preheat the air fryer oven to 355 degrees f.

4.In the air fryer oven pan, place lemongrass stalks. Cook for about 2-3 minutes. Remove the cashew mixture from air fryer and transfer into a bowl. Now, set the air fryer oven to 390 degrees f.

5.Place the chicken wings in air fryer pan. Cook for about 13-15 minutes further.

6.Transfer the wings into serving plates. Sprinkle with cashew mixture and serve.

Honey And Wine Chicken Breasts

Servings: 4

- 2 chicken breasts, rinsed and halved 1 tablespoon melted butter
- 1/2 teaspoon freshly ground pepper, or to taste 3/4 teaspoon sea salt, or to taste
- 1 teaspoon paprika
- 1 teaspoon dried rosemary
- **2** tablespoons dry white wine
- 1 tablespoon honey
- Firstly, pat the chicken breasts dry. Lightly coat them with the melted butter.
- Then, add the remaining .
- Transfer them to the air fryer basket; bake about 15 minutes at 330 degrees f°
- Serve warm and enjoy!

Chicken Fillets, Brie & Ham

Servings: 4

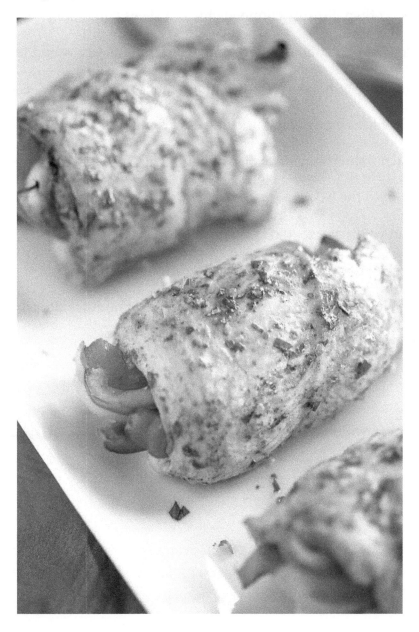

- 2 large chicken fillets Freshly ground black pepper

- 4 small slices of brie (or your cheese of choice)

- 1 tbsp. Freshly chopped chives 4 slices cured ham

1.Slice the fillets into four and make incisions as you would for a hamburger bun. Leave a little "hinge" uncut at the back. Season the inside and pop some brie and chives in there. Close them and wrap them each in a slice of ham. Brush with oil and pop them into the basket.

2.Heat your fryer to 350° f. Pour into the oven rack/basket. Place the rack on the middle-shelf of the air fryer oven.

3.Set temperature to 400°f and set time to 15 minutes. Roast the little parcels until they look tasty (15 min)

Bbq Chicken Recipe From Greece

Servings: 4

- 1 (8 ounce) container Fat-free plain yogurt2 tablespoons fresh lemon juice

- 2 teaspoons dried oregano

- 1-pound skinless, boneless chicken breast halves - cut into 1-inch pieces

- 1 large red onion, cut into wedges

- 1/2 teaspoon lemon zest 1/2 teaspoon salt

- large green bell pepper, cut into 1 1/2-inch pieces

- 1/3 cup crumbled feta cheese with basil and sun-dried tomatoes 1/4 teaspoon ground black pepper

- 1/4 teaspoon crushed dried rosemary
  In a shallow dish, mix well rosemary, pepper, salt, oregano, lemon juice, lemon zest, feta cheese, and yogurt. Add chicken and toss

- well to coat. Marinate in the ref for 3 hours.

- Thread bell pepper, onion, and chicken pieces in skewers. Place on skewer rack.

- For 12 minutes, cook on 360°f. Halfway through Cooking time, turnover skewers. If needed, cook in batches.
- Serve and enjoy.

Cheesy Chicken In Leek-Tomato Sauce

Servings: 4

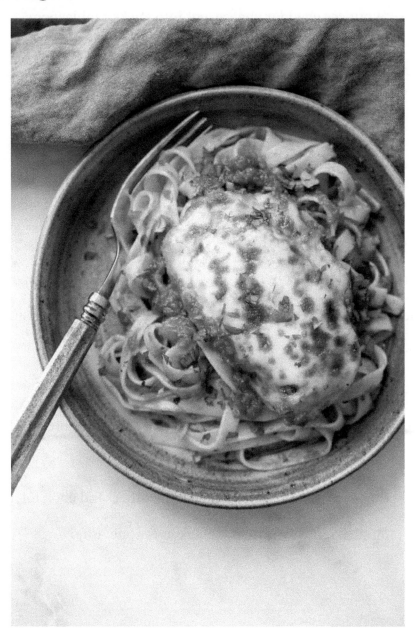

- 2 large-sized chicken breasts, cut in half lengthwise

- Salt and ground black pepper, to taste

- 4 ounces cheddar cheese, cut into sticks 1 tablespoon sesame oil

- 1cup leeks, chopped

- 2cloves garlic, minced

- 2/3 cup roasted vegetable stock 2/3 cup tomato puree

- 1teaspoon dried rosemary

- 1teaspoon dried thyme

1.Firstly, season chicken breasts with the salt and black pepper; place a piece of cheddar cheese in the middle. Then, tie it using a kitchen string; drizzle with sesame oil and reserve.

2.Add the leeks and garlic to the oven safe bowl.

3.Cook in the air fryer oven at 390 degrees f for 5 minutes or until tender.

4.Add the reserved chicken. Throw in the other and cook for 12 to 13 minutes more or until the chicken is done. Enjoy.

Oven Fried Chicken Wings

Servings: 3

- 1½ lbs. Chicken wings

- 1/3 c. Grated parmesan cheese

- 1/3 c. Breadcrumbs

- 1/8 tsp. Garlic powder

- 1/8 tsp. Onion powder

- ¼ c. Melted butter

- Salt and black pepper to taste

- Cooking spray

1.In a baking sheet, spray with Cooking spray.

2.A large bowl mix parmesan cheese, garlic powder, onion powder, black pepper, breadcrumbs and salt. Stir to combine well.

3.Dip chicken wings one at a time into melted butter and then into bread mixture until thoroughly covered. Arrange wings in single layer on the baking sheet.

4.Place on 1-inch rack and cook on high power (350 degrees f) for 10 minutes. Flip wings over and cook for another 10-12 minutes until no longer pink in center and juices run clear. Remove promptly from nuwave oven and serve.

Garlic Ginger Chicken Wings

Servings: 4

- 2pounds chicken wings

- 1 tbsp. Vegetable oil

- A pinch of salt and black pepper

- 1 tbsp. Frank's red-hot sauce 1/3 c. Flour

For Glaze

3 garlic cloves, minced

1 tbsp. Asian chili pepper sauce

¼ c. Rice wine vinegar 1 tbsp. Minced ginger

¼ c. Light brown Sugar 1½ tbsp. Soy sauce

- In a large mixing bowl, combine frank's red-hot sauce, vegetable oil, salt and pepper. Add chicken wings and toss to coat thoroughly.

- Place coated wings in large zip lock bag. Add flour, seal bag and shake until wings are coated with flour.

- Place wings on the 4-inch rack and cook on high power (350 degrees f) for 10 minutes. Turn wings over and cook for an additional 8 minutes.

- Meanwhile, in a large bowl, whisk together all for glaze. Place wings in glaze and toss to coat evenly. Place wings back on the 4-inch rack and cook on high power for an additional 5 minutes.

- Remove from oven then serve.

Apple-Stuffed Chicken Breast

Servings: 2

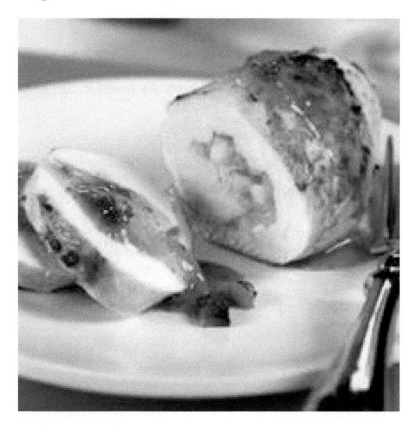

- 2chicken breasts

- 1large apple

- 1/4cup cheddar cheese, shredded

- 2 tbsp panko breadcrumbs

- 2tbsp. Chopped pecans,

- 2 tbsp. Light brown Sugar

- 1 tsp. Cinnamon

- 1tsp. Curry powder

1.In a large bowl, add chopped apple, cheese, breadcrumbs, pecans, brown Sugar, cinnamon, and curry powder. Stir to combine well.

2.Pound chicken breasts between waxed paper sheets till thick.

3.Spread half the apple mixture on every chicken breast. Roll the chicken up and secure with toothpicks.

4.Place chicken on the 4-inch rack and cook on high power for 12 minutes. Flip over and cook for another 10-12 minutes.

5.Serve hot.

Air Fried Turkey Breast

Servings: 6

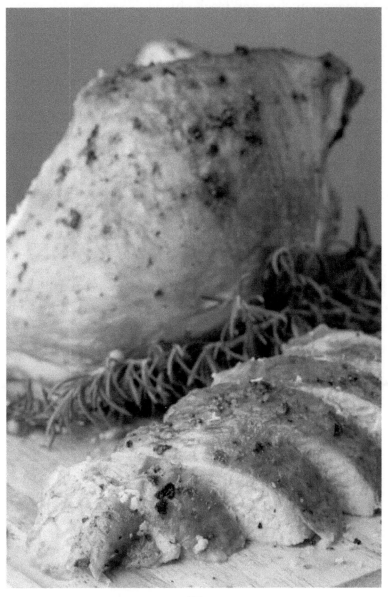

- 23/4 pounds turkey breast

- 2tablespoons unsalted butter

- 1tablespoon chopped fresh rosemary

- 1 teaspoon chopped fresh chives

- 1teaspoon minced fresh garlic

- 1/4 teaspoon black pepper

- 1/2teaspoon salt

- Preheat your air fryer toast oven to 350° f.

- In a bowl, mix chives, rosemary, garlic, salt and pepper until well combined. Cut in butter and mash until well blended.

- Rub the turkey breast with the herbed butter and then add to the air

- fryer toast oven basket; fry for 20 minutes. Turn the turkey breast and cook for another 20 minutes.

- Transfer the cooked turkey onto an aluminum foil and wrap; let rest for at least 10 minutes and then slice it up. Serve warm.

Healthy Turkey Lettuce Wraps

Servings: 4

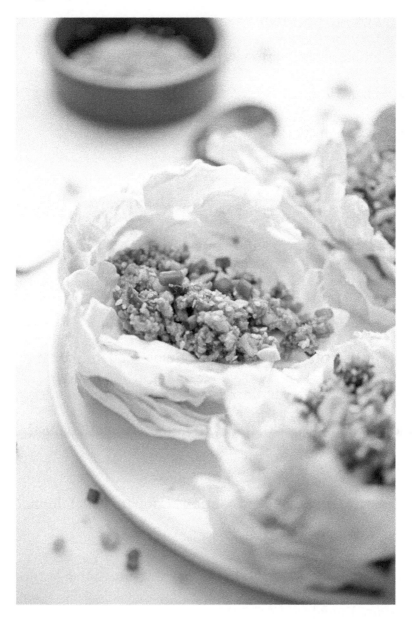

- 250g ground turkey

- 1/2 small onion, finely chopped

- 1 garlic clove, minced

- 2tablespoons extra virgin olive oil

- 1 head lettuce

- teaspoon cumin

- 1/2tablespoon fresh ginger, sliced

- 2 tablespoons apple cider vinegar

- 2tablespoons freshly chopped cilantro

- 1 teaspoon freshly ground black pepper

- 1 teaspoon sea salt

1.Sauté garlic and onion in extra virgin olive oil until fragrant and translucent in your air fryer toast oven pan at 350 degrees f.

2.Add turkey and cook well for 5-8 minutes or until done to desire.

3.Add in the remaining and continue Cooking for 5 minutes more.

4.To serve, spoon a spoonful of turkey mixture onto a lettuce leaf and wrap. Enjoy!

Duo Crisp Chicken Wings

Servings: 6

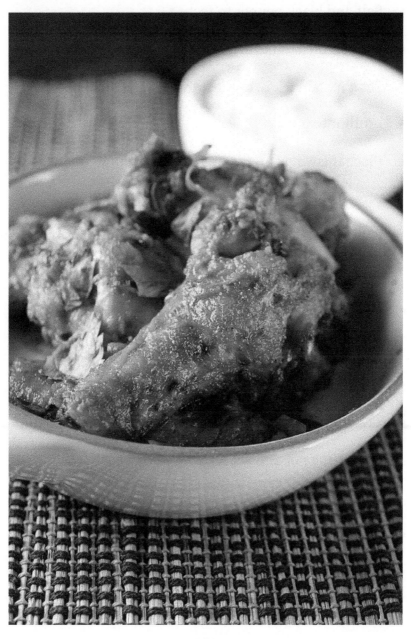

- 12chicken wings

- 1/2 cup chicken broth

- Salt and black pepper to taste

- 1/4 cup melted butter

- Set a metal rack in the instant pot duo crisp and pour broth into it.

- Place the wings on the metal rack then put on its pressure-Cooking lid.

- Hit the "pressure button" and select 8 minutes of Cooking time, then press "start."

- Once the instant pot duo beeps, do a quick release and remove its

- lid.

- Transfer the pressure-cooked wings to a plate.

- Empty the pot and set an air fryer basket in the instant pot duo

- Toss the wings with butter and seasoning.

- Spread the seasoned wings in the air fryer basket.

- Put on the air fryer lid, hit the air fryer button, and then set the time to 10 minutes.10. Remove the lid and serve.
- Enjoy!

Italian Whole Chicken

Servings: 4

- 1whole chicken

- 2tablespoon or spray of oil of choice

- 1teaspoon garlic powder 1 teaspoon onion powder
  1teaspoon paprika

- 1teaspoon italian seasoning

- 2tablespoon montreal steak seasoning

- 1.5cup chicken broth

- Whisk all the seasoning in a bowl and rub it on the
  chicken.

- Set a metal rack in the instant pot duo crisp and pour
  broth into it.

- Place the chicken on the metal rack then put on its
  pressure- Cooking lid.

- Hit the "pressure button" and select 25 minutes of
  Cooking time, then press "start."

- Once the instant pot duo beeps, do a natural release and
  remove its lid.

- Transfer the pressure-cooked chicken to a plate.

- Empty the pot and set an air fryer basket in the instant pot duo.

- Toss the chicken pieces with oil to coat well.

- Spread the seasoned chicken in the air fryer basket.

- Put on the air fryer lid, hit the air fryer button, and then set the time to 10 minutes.

- Remove the lid and serve. Enjoy!

Chicken Pot Pie

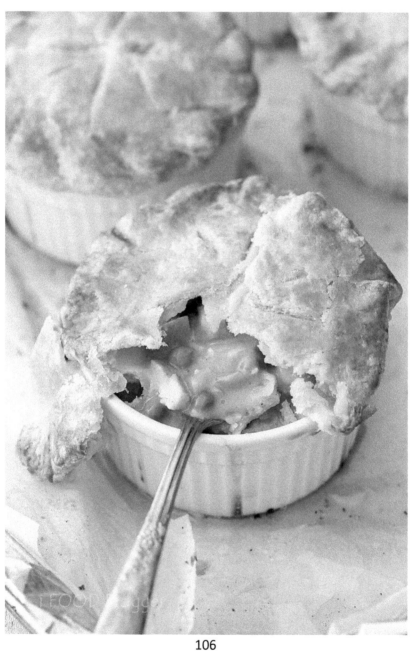

- 2tbsp olive oil

- 1-pound chicken breast cubed

- 1 tbsp garlic powder

- 1tbsp thyme

- 1tbsp pepper

- 1cup chicken broth

- 12oz. Bag frozen mixed vegetables

- 4 large potatoes cubed

- 10oz. Can cream of chicken soup

- 1cup heavy cream 1 pie crust

- 1egg

- 1tbsp water

- Hit sauté on the instant pot duo crispy and add chicken and olive oil.

- Sauté chicken for 5 minutes then stirs in spices.

- Pour in the broth along with vegetables and cream of chicken soup

- Put on the pressure-Cooking lid and seal it.

- Hit the "pressure button" and select 10 minutes of Cooking time, then press "start."
- Once the instant pot duo beeps, do a quick release and remove its lid.
- Remove the lid and stir in cream.
- Hit sauté and cook for 2 minutes.
- Enjoy!

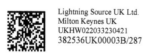

Lightning Source UK Ltd.
Milton Keynes UK
UKHW022033230421
382536UK00003B/287

9 781801 455855